FATTY LIVER COOKBOOK FOR SENIORS

Detoxify and Revitalize Your Body with Nutritious Recipes That Will Help Increase Energy and Ignite Vitality

Nancy J. Atkins.

The doctor's words hung heavy in the air, a leaden echo against the sterile white walls. "Fatty liver disease," he'd announced, his pronouncement stealing the vibrant hues from my friend's face. John, a man whose laughter had seasoned countless conversations, now stared silently at the table, his appetite, once as robust as his humor, as shriveled as a discarded autumn leaf.

John wasn't just a friend; he was a testament to life's boisterous symphony. A chef by passion, his kitchen was a stage where flavors pirouetted, aromas were conducted, and plates became canvases for culinary masterpieces. Yet this invisible foe had silenced his culinary concerto, replacing vibrant spices with the bitter notes of fatigue and disquiet.

But John, ever the maestro, refused to surrender. He wouldn't be reduced to a passive audience in his own health story. Armed with a steely resolve and a hunger for reclaiming his zest for life, he embarked on a culinary odyssey, not into exotic lands but into the heart of his own kitchen. This wasn't about deprivation, but about a meticulous composition of taste and health, a culinary score he would orchestrate himself.

This book is a testament to John's triumph, a cookbook not just for seniors battling fatty liver disease but for anyone seeking to harmonize well-being with the pleasure of delicious food. It's a symphony of scientifically guided recipes, each note carefully chosen to nourish the body and tantalize the taste buds. Forget restrictive, joyless diets. This is a culinary crescendo, an allegro of vibrant Mediterranean flavors, whispered wisdom from forgotten kitchens, and the subtle but powerful harmony of modern nutritional science.

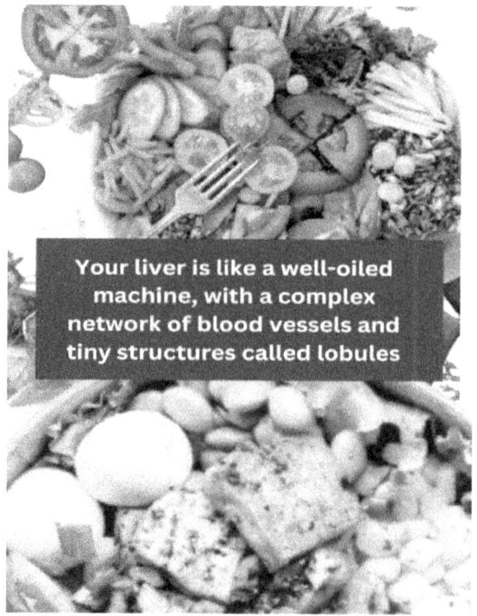

CHAPTER 1

Your Liver: The Unsung Hero of Your Body

The liver, nestled beneath your ribs on the right side of your abdomen, is a silent powerhouse. Though often overlooked, this reddish-brown organ plays a vital role in keeping you healthy and functioning. It's like a tireless factory, constantly working behind the scenes to perform over 500 essential tasks, making it one of the most important organs in your body.

What does your liver do?

Think of your liver as a multi-talented performer, juggling several critical roles:

- **Filtration:** Your liver acts as a natural filter, removing toxins and waste products from your blood. This includes everything from medications and alcohol to bacteria and excess hormones.

- **Metabolism:** It's the master chef of your body, processing nutrients from your food and converting them into energy or storing them for later use. This includes breaking down carbohydrates for sugar, fats for energy, and proteins for building and repairing tissues.

- **Production:** The liver is a prolific manufacturer, producing essential substances like cholesterol (needed for cell membranes and hormones), bile (which helps digest fats), and proteins that help blood clot and fight infections.

- **Storage:** It's a well-stocked pantry, storing important nutrients like vitamins A, D, E, K, and B12, as well as iron and sugar, for when your body needs them.

- **Regulation:** Your liver acts as a control center, regulating your blood sugar levels, cholesterol levels, and hormone production. This helps maintain internal balance and keeps your body functioning smoothly.

How does your liver work?

Your liver is like a well-oiled machine, with a complex network of blood vessels and tiny structures called lobules.

Here's a simplified look at its operation:

1. **Blood arrives:** Blood from your digestive tract, carrying nutrients and toxins, enters the liver through the portal vein.

2. **Filtration begins: liver** cells, called hepatocytes, filter the blood, removing toxins and waste products.

3. **Nutrient processing:** Nutrients are extracted from the blood and processed for storage or use.

4. **Bile production:** Bile, a greenish fluid that helps digest fats, is produced in the liver and stored in the gallbladder.

5. **Waste disposal:** Toxins and waste products are either sent back to the bloodstream to be excreted through the kidneys or packaged into bile and sent to the intestines for elimination.

6. **Regulation:** The liver monitors various levels in your body, like blood sugar and cholesterol, and adjusts its functions accordingly to maintain balance.

Your liver is like the conductor of an orchestra, ensuring all your other organs play their part in harmony. Here are just a few examples of how your organs depend on your liver:

- **Brain:** Your liver helps remove toxins that can damage brain cells and regulates blood sugar levels, which are crucial for brain function.

- **Heart:** The liver helps regulate cholesterol levels, preventing fatty buildup in the arteries and reducing the risk of heart disease.

- **Kidneys:** The liver helps break down and remove waste products, reducing the burden on your kidneys.

- **Bones:** The liver stores and activates vitamin D, which is essential for bone health.

- **Immune system:** The liver produces proteins that help fight infections and inflammation.

A healthy liver is essential for general well-being. Here are some tips:

- **Eat a balanced diet: choose** plenty of fruits, vegetables, and whole grains, and limit saturated fat, processed foods, and sugary drinks.

- **Maintain a healthy weight.** Excess weight can put stress on your liver.

- **Limit alcohol: excessive** alcohol consumption can damage liver cells.

- **Get regular exercise.** Physical activity helps your body process nutrients and toxins more efficiently.

- **Avoid toxins:** Limit your exposure to environmental toxins and harmful chemicals.

- **Get regular check-ups.** Your doctor can monitor your liver health through blood tests and physical exams.

By understanding your liver's vital role and taking steps to keep it healthy, you can ensure it continues to conduct the symphony of your well-being for years to come.

Your liver's influence extends beyond its own walls, composing the rhythm of your health in a delicate interplay with other vital organs. Let's delve deeper into this intricate musical score, exploring the liver's vital connections to your heart, brain, and even your emotional well-being.

Liver and Heart: A Duet in Rhythm

Imagine your liver and heart as two musicians, their melodies intertwining in a harmonious tango. The liver, like a diligent percussionist, regulates cholesterol levels, keeping your arteries clear and ensuring smooth blood flow to the heart. This reduces the strain on your heart muscle and lowers your risk of heart disease, a silent predator lurking in the shadows of unhealthy livers. Conversely, a healthy heart pumps blood efficiently, delivering vital oxygen and nutrients to the liver and fueling its tireless metabolic processes. This synchronized performance keeps your cardiovascular system humming in perfect rhythm.

The liver and brain are not just physical neighbors but partners in an intricate ballet of cognitive function. The liver detoxifies the blood, removing harmful chemicals that can impair brain function and memory. It also regulates blood sugar levels, providing a steady stream of energy for your neurons to fire and synapses to connect. When the liver falters, this delicate balance can be disrupted, leading to fatigue, brain fog, and even dementia. But nourish your liver with a healthy diet, and you nourish your mind, fostering a vibrant symphony of thought and clarity.

Hormones and Emotions: The Conductor's Baton

The liver plays a masterful role in conducting your hormonal orchestra. It metabolizes and breaks down hormones, maintaining the delicate balance that governs your mood, energy, and even libido. When your liver is sluggish, this hormonal equilibrium can be thrown into disarray. Excess estrogen, for example, can lead to anxiety, mood swings, and even depression. Conversely, a well-functioning liver ensures smooth hormonal flow, keeping your emotions in tune and your spirit buoyant.

By nurturing your liver, you don't just protect a single organ; you safeguard the entire orchestra of your well-being. Every bite you choose becomes a note in the symphony, and every healthy habit becomes a verse in the song of your health. So, listen to your body, nourish your liver, and let the vibrant melody of well-being resonate throughout your life. Remember, the conductor's baton lies in your hands, and the power to compose a harmonious health symphony is yours.

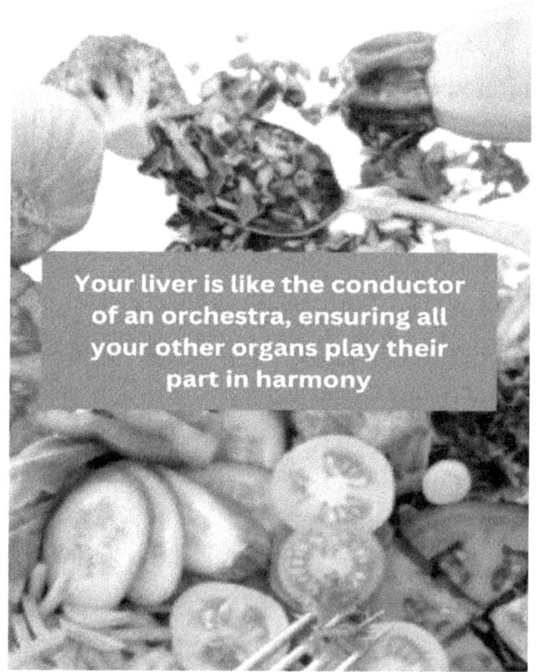

CHAPTER 2

Fatty Liver: A Closer Look

The liver, the body's silent superhero, conducts approximately 500 vital functions, including toxin removal and protein production. However, if this unsung hero begins to accumulate excess fat, he or she may develop fatty liver disease. Let's look at the various sorts, their worldwide impact, and the special connection to pregnancy.

Different types of fatty liver

Nonalcoholic Fatty Liver Disease (NAFLD) is the most common form, affecting 25% of adults globally. NAFLD occurs in two stages:

> Simple fatty liver refers to excess fat storage in the liver without inflammation or injury.

> Nonalcoholic steatohepatitis (NASH) causes fat accumulation, inflammation, and liver cell destruction. NASH can develop into fibrosis (scarring) and even cirrhosis (severe liver damage).

AFLD (Alcoholic Fatty Liver Disease) is caused by excessive alcohol consumption. AFLD, like NAFLD, proceeds in phases, potentially leading to cirrhosis.

The Global Fatty Liver Phenomenon

Fatty liver disease is a global health issue that affects people of all ages and races. Several reasons contribute to the rise:

Lifestyle changes: obesity and insulin resistance, which are risk factors for NAFLD, are caused by increased consumption of processed foods and sugary drinks, as well as decreased physical activity.

Westernized diet: The Western diet, high in saturated fat and processed carbohydrates, contributes to the fatty liver epidemic. Environmental variables, such as exposure to chemicals and pollution, can significantly raise the risk of the condition.

Pregnancy can be a challenging time for the body, including the liver. While some expecting moms experience a brief fatty liver disease as a result of hormonal changes, this normally recovers after childbirth. However, pre-existing NAFLD might develop during pregnancy, raising the risk of problems for both the mother and the child.

Effective management of fatty liver disease requires early diagnosis and lifestyle changes. Maintaining a healthy weight, eating a balanced diet rich in fruits, vegetables, and whole grains, and engaging in regular exercise are all important for preventing and treating the illness. In severe situations, medicines or even a liver transplant may be required.

Food to Eat For Fatty Liver

Foods recommended for fatty liver disease include berries, broccoli, spinach, leafy greens, and cruciferous vegetables. High in antioxidants and fiber to protect the liver and prevent inflammation.

- Choose whole grains such as oats, brown rice, quinoa, and whole-wheat bread instead of processed grains. High in fiber and minerals to help control blood sugar and insulin levels.

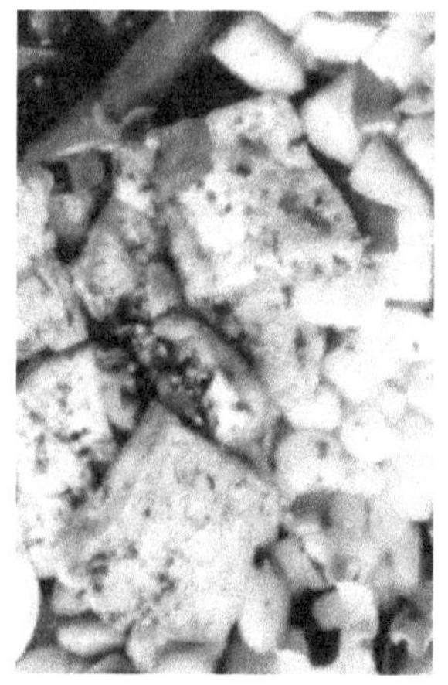

Avocados, nuts, seeds, olive oil, and fatty fish include beneficial fats that lower inflammation and improve cholesterol levels.

- Foods high in lean protein include fish, chicken, beans, and lentils. Avoid processed and red meats that are high in saturated fat and cholesterol.

- Moderate coffee consumption (1-3 cups per day) can improve liver health. • Green tea contains antioxidants that protect the liver from harm.

Foods to Avoid for Fatty Liver Disease

- Limit fructose-rich beverages such as soda, juice, and sports drinks to avoid the risk of fatty liver disease.

- Avoid refined carbs such as white bread, spaghetti, and rice. These foods can trigger blood sugar surges, which put strain on your liver.

- Fried foods are high in harmful fats that can lead to fatty liver disease.

- Processed meats, such as sausage, bacon, and hot dogs, have high levels of saturated fat and sodium, which can affect your liver.

- Excess alcohol consumption is a significant risk factor for fatty liver disease. If you have alcohol, avoid it altogether.

Meats to Consume For Fatty Liver Disease

- Fatty fish such as salmon, sardines, tuna, and mackerel contain omega-3 fatty acids, which can reduce inflammation and enhance liver health.

- Skinless chicken and turkey are lean protein sources with low saturated fat and cholesterol, making them suitable for individuals with fatty liver disease.

- Beans and lentils provide plant-based protein and fiber, which are healthy for liver function.

- Limit consumption of red meat, such as beef and pork, to once or twice a week due to its high saturated fat content.

- Avoid processed meats such as sausage, bacon, and hot dogs because of their high saturated fat and sodium content, which is damaging to the liver.

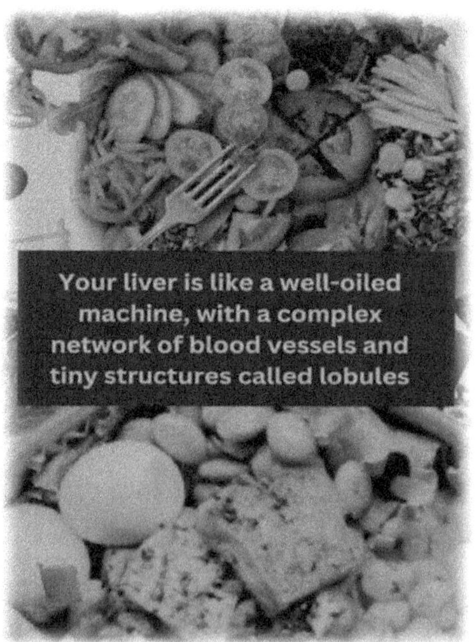

CHAPTER 3

Delicious Breakfast Recipes

Oatmeal with Fresh Berries:

Cooking Time: 10–15 minutes

Ingredients:

- 1/2 cup rolled oats
- Use 1 cup of milk of your choice (dairy, almond, coconut, etc.).
- Optional: 1/4 cup water (modify to desired consistency).
- 1/4 cup fresh berries (blueberries, raspberries, strawberries)
- Optional: add 1 tablespoon of honey or maple syrup.

Instructions:

1. Combine oats, milk, and water (if using) in a saucepan. Bring to a boil, then reduce heat and simmer for 5–10 minutes, stirring occasionally, until the oats are tender and creamy.
2. Remove from heat and stir in fresh berries, honey or maple syrup (if using), and cinnamon.
3. Serve warm, topped with additional berries and nuts (optional).

Nutritional Value (per serving, with dairy milk and no added honey or syrup):

- Calories: 250
- Protein: 7g
- Fat: 4g
- Carbohydrates: 40g
- Fiber: 4g

Veggie and Mushroom Scramble:

Cooking Time: 15-20 minutes

Ingredients:

- 2 eggs
- 1/2 cup chopped vegetables of your choice (bell peppers, onions, spinach, etc.)
- 1/4 cup sliced mushrooms
- 1/4 cup of milk of your choice
- 1 tablespoon of olive oil
- Salt and pepper to taste
- Optional toppings: shredded cheese, avocado slices, hot sauce

Instructions:

1. Whisk the eggs and milk together in a bowl.
2. You need to heat olive oil in a skillet over medium heat. Sauté vegetables and mushrooms until softened, about 5 minutes.

3. Pour in the egg mixture and cook, stirring occasionally, until scrambled to your desired consistency.
4. For taste, season with salt and pepper.
5. Serve warm, topped with the desired toppings.

Nutritional Value (per serving, with dairy milk and no added cheese):

- Calories: 200
- Protein: 12g
- Fat: 10g
- Carbohydrates: 5g

Blueberry Almond Overnight Oats:

Cooking Time: Overnight (approximately 8 hours)

Ingredients:

- 1/2 cup rolled oats
- 1/2 cup of milk of your choice
- 1/4 cup yogurt (Greek or dairy-free)
- 1/4 cup fresh or frozen blueberries
- 1 tablespoon of chia seeds
- 1 tablespoon of honey or maple syrup
- 1/4 teaspoon almond extract
- 1/4 cup chopped almonds

Instructions:

1. 1. Mix every ingredient in a container or
    basin. Stir thoroughly to ensure that
    everything is combined.
2. Cover and refrigerate overnight.
3. In the morning, stir before serving, and top
    with additional berries and almonds
    (optional).

Nutritional Value (per serving, with dairy milk and
yogurt):

- Calories: 350
- Protein: 15g
- Fat: 15g
- Carbohydrates: 40g
- Fiber: 6g

Banana Walnut Muffins:

Cooking Time: 20–25 minutes

Ingredients:

- 1 1/2 cups mashed, ripe bananas
- 1/3 cup melted butter or coconut oil
- 1 egg
- 1/2 cup of milk of your choice
- 1 1/2 cups whole wheat flour
- 1/2 cup unbleached all-purpose flour
- 1 teaspoon baking powder
- 1/2 teaspoon baking soda

- 1/4 teaspoon salt
- 1/2 cup chopped walnuts
- 1/4 cup brown sugar (optional)

Instructions:

1. Preheat the oven to 375°F (190°C). Then line a muffin tin with paper liners.
2. In a large bowl, combine mashed bananas, melted butter, eggs, and milk. Stir until well combined.
3. In a separate bowl, whisk together the dry ingredients (flours, baking powder, baking soda, and salt).
4. Add dry ingredients to wet ingredients and fold in gently until just combined. Do not over mix.
5. Fold in chopped walnuts and brown sugar (if using).
6. Divide the batter evenly among the muffin cups.
7. Bake for 20–25 minutes, or until a toothpick inserted into the center comes out clean.
8. Let cool in the pan for a few minutes before transferring to a wire rack to

Cooking Time: Approximately 10–15 minutes

Ingredients:

- 2 large eggs
- 1/4 cup chopped vegetables of your choice (e.g., onions, peppers, mushrooms, spinach)
- 1 tablespoon of olive oil
- 1/4 cup shredded cheese (optional)
- Salt and pepper to taste

Instructions:

1. Whisk the eggs together in a bowl with a fork until light and frothy.
2. Warm the olive oil in a nonstick skillet over medium heat. Cook the chopped vegetables until softened, about 5 minutes.
3. Pour the egg mixture into the pan and tilt the pan to spread the eggs evenly.
4. Season with salt and pepper.
5. Once the bottom of the omelet is set, gently fold one half over the other using a spatula.
6. If using cheese, sprinkle it over the top of the omelet and let it melt for another minute.
7. Serve immediately.

Nutritional Value: (per serving, without cheese)

- Calories: 160
- Protein: 12g

- Fat: 8g
- Carbohydrates: 1g

Pineapple Macha and Beet Chia Pudding

Cooking Time: Overnight (approximately 8 hours)

Ingredients:

- 1/2 cup chia seeds
- 1 cup unsweetened almond milk or coconut milk
- 1/2 cup chopped pineapple
- 1/4 cup cooked and mashed beetroot
- 1 teaspoon of matcha powder
- 1/2 teaspoon honey or maple syrup (optional)
- Granola and fresh fruit (optional, for topping)

Instructions:

1. In a jar or bowl, combine chia seeds, almond milk, pineapple, beetroot, matcha powder, and honey (if using). Stir well to combine.
2. Cover and refrigerate overnight.
3. In the morning, stir the pudding again and top with granola and fresh fruit, if desired.

Nutritional Value: (per serving)

- Calories: 250
- Protein: 5g

- Fat: 12g
- Carbohydrates: 30g

Cooking Time: Approximately 30 minutes

Ingredients:

- 1/2 cup tapioca pearls
- 4 cups milk of your choice (e.g., dairy, almond, coconut)
- 1/4 cup sugar
- 1/4 teaspoon vanilla extract
- Pinch of salt

Instructions:

1. In a saucepan, combine the tapioca pearls, milk, sugar, vanilla extract, and salt. Bring to a boil over medium heat while stirring regularly.
2. Reduce the heat to low and simmer for 20–25 minutes, stirring occasionally, until the tapioca pearls are translucent and the mixture thickens.
3. Remove from heat and allow to cool before serving.
4. You can serve the pudding warm or chilled.

Nutritional Value: (per serving, with dairy milk)

- Calories: 250

- Protein: 5g
- Fat: 8g
- Carbohydrates: 40g

Breakfast Taco

Cooking Time: Approximately 10 minutes

Ingredients:

- 2 tortillas of your choice (e.g., corn, flour, whole wheat)
- Scrambled eggs or tofu scramble
- Black beans or pinto beans
- Avocado slices
- Salsa
- Optional toppings: cheese, cilantro, hot sauce, pickled onions

Instructions:

1. Warm the tortillas according to the package instructions.
2. Scramble the eggs or prepare the tofu scramble.
3. Spread the beans on the tortillas.
4. Top with scrambled eggs, avocado slices, salsa, and any other desired toppings.
5. Fold the tortillas and enjoy!

Nutritional Value: (per serving)

- Calories: 300-400 (varies depending on ingredients)
- Protein: 15-20g
- Fat: 10-15g
- Carbohydrates: 30-40g

Buckwheat and Grapefruit Porridge

Cooking Time: Approximately 15 minutes

Ingredients:

- 1/2 cup buckwheat groats
- 1 cup of water or your desired milk
- 1/2 grapefruit, segmented
- 1 tablespoon of honey or maple syrup
- 1/4 teaspoon cinnamon
- Pinch of salt

Instructions:

1. In a saucepan, bring the water or milk to a boil. Reduce the heat to low while you add the buckwheat groats. Simmer for 10–15 minutes, or until the groats are tender and most of the liquid has been absorbed.
2. Remove from heat and stir in the grapefruit segments, honey, or maple.
3. Season with cinnamon and salt to taste.
4. Serve immediately.

Nutritional Value: (per serving, with water)

- Calories: 250
- Protein: 5g
- Fat: 7g
- Carbohydrates: 40g

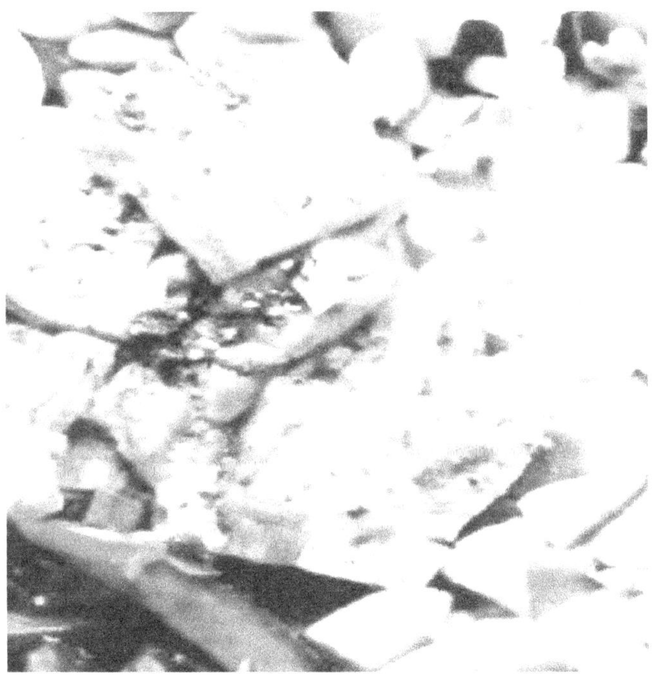

CHAPTER 4

Crains, Legumes, and Beans

Kidney Beans and Beet Salad:

Cooking Time: 20 minutes (plus cooling time)

Ingredients:

- 1 15-ounce can of kidney beans, drained and rinsed
- 2 medium beets, roasted and cubed
- 1/2 red onion, thinly sliced
- 1/4 cup crumbled feta cheese
- 2 tablespoons chopped fresh parsley
- 2 tablespoons of olive oil
- 1 tablespoon of lemon juice
- Salt and pepper to taste

Instructions:

1. In a large bowl, combine kidney beans, beets, and red onion.
2. In a separate bowl, whisk together the olive oil, lemon juice, salt, and pepper.
3. Pour the dressing over the bean mixture and toss to coat.
4. Top with crumbled feta cheese and fresh parsley.

5. Serve immediately, or chill for 30 minutes
   for even deeper flavors.

Nutritional Value (per serving):

- Calories: 250
- Protein: 10g
- Fat: 10g
- Carbohydrates: 30g
- Fiber: 5g

Black Eyed Peas Stew:

Cooking Time: 45 minutes

Ingredients:

- 1 tablespoon of olive oil
- 1 onion, chopped
- 2 cloves garlic, minced
- 1 green bell pepper, chopped
- 1 red bell pepper, chopped
- 1 15-ounce can of diced tomatoes
- 4 cups of vegetable broth
- 1 15-ounce can of black-eyed peas, drained and rinsed
- 1 cup chopped kale or spinach
- 1 teaspoon dried thyme
- 1/2 teaspoon smoked paprika
- Salt and pepper to taste

Instructions:

1. 1. Warm olive oil in a big pot over medium heat. Cook for 5 minutes, or until the onion has softened.
2. Add garlic and bell peppers, and cook for another 5 minutes.
3. Stir in diced tomatoes, vegetable broth, black-eyed peas, kale or spinach, thyme, and paprika. Season with salt and pepper.
4. Bring to a boil, then reduce heat and simmer for 30 minutes, or until thickened.
5. Serve warm with crusty bread or rice.

Nutritional Value (per serving):

- Calories: 300
- Protein: 15g
- Fat: 5g
- Carbohydrates: 40g
- Fiber: 8g

Kidney Beans and Parsley-Lemon Salad:

Cooking Time: 10 minutes

Ingredients:

- 1 15-ounce can of kidney beans, drained and rinsed
- 1/2 cup chopped fresh parsley
- 1/4 cup chopped red onion

- 2 tablespoons of olive oil
- 1 tablespoon of lemon juice
- Salt and pepper to taste

Instructions:

1. In a large bowl, combine kidney beans, parsley, and red onion.
2. In a separate bowl, whisk together the olive oil, lemon juice, salt, and pepper.
3. Pour the dressing over the bean mixture and toss to coat.
4. Serve immediately as a side dish or on top of salads.

Nutritional Value (per serving):

- Calories: 150
- Protein: 8g
- Fat: 5g
- Carbohydrates: 20g
- Fiber: 4g

Chickpea Alfredo Sauce:

Cooking Time: 20 minutes

Ingredients:

- 1 15-ounce can of chickpeas, drained and rinsed
- 1/2 cup cashews, soaked for at least 2 hours or overnight

- 1/4 cup nutritional yeast
- 1/4 cup of water
- 2 tablespoons of lemon juice
- 2 cloves garlic, minced
- 1/2 teaspoon dried oregano
- Salt and pepper to taste

Instructions:

1. In a high-powered blender, combine chickpeas, cashews, nutritional yeast, water, lemon juice, garlic, and oregano. Blend until smooth and creamy.
2. You have to season with salt and pepper to taste.
3. Use this sauce over pasta, vegetables, or as a dip.

Nutritional Value (per serving):

- Calories: 200
- Protein: 10g
- Fat: 10g
- Carbohydrates: 20g

- Fiber: 5g

Italian White Bean Soup:

Cooking Time: 45 minutes

Ingredients:

- 1 tablespoon of olive oil
- 1 onion, chopped
- 2 cloves garlic, minced
- 1 carrot, chopped
- 1 celery stalk, chopped
- 4 cups of vegetable broth
- 1 15-ounce can of cannellini beans, drained and rinsed
- 1 15-oz can pinto beans, drained and rinsed
- 1 14.5-oz can diced tomatoes, undrained
- 1 tablespoon chopped fresh parsley
- 1/2 teaspoon dried oregano
- Salt and pepper to taste

Instructions:

1. Warm olive oil in a big pot on medium heat. Cook until the onion softens, which should take around 5 minutes.
2. Add garlic, carrot, and celery, and cook for another 5 minutes.
3. Stir in vegetable broth, cannellini beans, pinto beans, diced tomatoes with their juices, parsley, and oregano. Season with salt and pepper.
4. Bring to a boil, then reduce heat and simmer for 30 minutes, or until thickened.
5. Serve warm with crusty bread or a side salad.

Nutritional Value (per serving):

- Calories: 300
- Protein: 15g
- Fat: 5g
- Carbohydrates: 40g
- Fiber: 8g

Chickpea Eggplant Salad:

Cooking Time: 20 minutes (plus cooling time)

Ingredients:

- 1 large eggplant, cubed
- 1 tablespoon of olive oil
- 1/2 red onion, finely chopped
- 1 can (15 oz) chickpeas, drained and rinsed
- 1/2 cup chopped fresh parsley
- 1/4 cup crumbled feta cheese (optional)
- 2 tablespoons of lemon juice
- 1 tablespoon of olive oil
- Salt and pepper to taste

Instructions:

1. Preheat the oven to 400°F (200°C). Toss eggplant cubes with olive oil and spread on a baking sheet. Roast for 15-20 minutes, or until tender and golden brown.
2. While the eggplant roasts, finely chop the red onion.

3. In a large bowl, combine roasted eggplant, chickpeas, red onion, and parsley.
4. In a small bowl, whisk together the lemon juice, olive oil, salt, and pepper. Drizzle over the chickpea mixture and toss to coat.
5. Top with crumbled feta cheese (optional) and serve immediately, or chill for 30 minutes for deeper flavors.

Nutritional Value (per serving):

- Calories: 250
- Protein: 8g
- Fat: 10g
- Carbohydrates: 30g
- Fiber: 5g

Sicilian Style Zoodle Spaghetti:

Cooking Time: 30 minutes

Ingredients:

- 4 large zucchini, spiralized into zoodles
- 1 tablespoon of olive oil
- 1/2 red onion, finely chopped
- 2 cloves garlic, minced
- 1 can (28 oz) of diced tomatoes, undrained
- 1/2 cup chopped fresh basil
- 1/4 cup chopped fresh parsley

- 1 teaspoon dried oregano
- Salt and pepper to taste

Instructions:

1. Heat olive oil in a large skillet over medium heat. Add the red onion to it and cook until softened, which should take about 5 minutes.
2. Stir in the garlic and cook for another minute, until fragrant.
3. Add diced tomatoes with their juices, basil, parsley, oregano, salt, and pepper. While boiling it, reduce the heat and simmer for 15 minutes.
4. Meanwhile, spiralize the zucchini into zoodles using a spiralizer or julienne peeler.
5. Add zoodles to the simmering sauce and cook for 5-7 minutes, or until tender but still with a slight bite.
6. Serve immediately, garnished with additional fresh basil and parsley (optional).

Nutritional Value (per serving):

- Calories: 200
- Protein: 5g
- Fat: 5g
- Carbohydrates: 35g
- Fiber: 5g

Cooking Time: 10 minutes (plus soaking time for beans)

Ingredients:

- 1 cup dried chickpeas, soaked overnight and drained
- 1/2 cup frozen peas
- 1/4 cup packed with fresh cilantro leaves
- 2 tablespoons of tahini
- 2 tablespoons of lemon juice
- 1 clove garlic, minced
- 1/4 cup olive oil
- Salt and pepper to taste

Instructions:

1. Combine drained chickpeas, peas, cilantro, tahini, lemon juice, garlic, and olive oil in a food processor.
2. Process until smooth and creamy, scraping down the sides as needed.
3. You have to season with salt and pepper to taste.
4. Hummus can be enjoyed immediately or stored in an airtight container in the refrigerator for up to 5 days.

Nutritional Value (per serving):

- Calories: 200
- Protein: 8g
- Fat: 8g
- Carbohydrates: 20g
- Fiber: 5g

Spaghetti, Lemon, Avocado, and White Sauce:

Cooking Time: 15 minutes

Ingredients:

- 1 ripe avocado, peeled and pitted
- 1/2 cup raw cashews, soaked for at least 2 hours or overnight
- 1/4 cup of water
- 1/4 cup of lemon juice
- 2 cloves garlic, minced
- 1/4 cup nutritional yeast
- Salt and pepper to taste

Instructions:

1. Combine all ingredients in a high-powered blender and blend until smooth and creamy.
2. Season with salt and pepper, to taste.

3. Toss cooked spaghetti with the sauce and serve immediately with desired toppings such as cherry tomatoes, fresh basil, or roasted vegetables.

Nutritional Value (per serving):

- Calories: 300
- 5. Fennel Wild Rice Risotto:
- Cooking Time: 45 minutes
- Ingredients:
- 1 tablespoon of olive oil
- 1/2 onion, finely chopped
- 1 bulb of fennel, thinly sliced
- 1 clove garlic, minced
- 1 cup wild rice, rinsed
- 4 cups of vegetable broth
- 1/2 cup dry white wine (optional)
- 1/4 cup grated Parmesan cheese
- Salt and pepper to taste

Instructions:

- Warm olive oil in a big pot over medium heat. Cook until the onion has softened, which should take around 5 minutes.
- Stir in the fennel and cook for another 5 minutes, until softened and slightly golden brown.

- Then add garlic and cook for 1 minute, until fragrant.
- Stir in the wild rice and cook for another minute, coating the grains with the oil and aromatics.
- Pour in white wine (optional) and simmer until evaporated, about 2 minutes.
- Add vegetable broth, 1/2 cup at a time, stirring constantly until each addition is absorbed before adding the next. This process will take approximately 30–35 minutes.
- Once the rice is tender and creamy, stir in Parmesan cheese and season with salt and pepper to taste.
- Serve immediately, garnished with additional Parmesan cheese and fresh herbs (optional).
- Nutritional Value (per serving):
- Calories: 350
- Protein: 8g
- Fat: 10g
- Carbohydrates: 50g
- Fiber: 5g

CHAPTER 5

Pork, Beef, and Lamb: Hearty Meat Delights

Hot Pork Meatballs:

Cooking Time: 40 minutes (including baking)

Ingredients:

- 1/2 lb. ground pork
- 1/2 cup of breadcrumbs
- 1/4 cup of milk
- 1 egg, beaten
- 1/2 onion, finely chopped
- 1 clove garlic, minced
- 1/2 teaspoon dried oregano
- 1/4 teaspoon salt
- 1/4 teaspoon black pepper
- 1/4 cup tomato sauce
- 1/4 cup of water

Instructions:

1. Preheat the oven to 375°F (190°C). Line a baking sheet with parchment paper.
2. In a large bowl, combine ground pork, breadcrumbs, milk, egg, onion, garlic,

oregano, salt, and pepper. Mix well until
evenly combined.

3. Form the mixture into meatballs, about 1
    inch in diameter. Place it on the prepared
    baking sheet.
4. In a small bowl, whisk together the tomato
    sauce and water. Pour over the meatballs.
5. Bake for 25–30 minutes, or until meatballs
    are cooked through and browned.
6. Serve hot with your favorite dipping sauce
    or on pasta.

Nutritional Value (per serving, without dipping
sauce):

- Calories: 300
- Protein: 25g
- Fat: 15g
- Carbohydrates: 20g
- Fiber: 1g

Pork and Peas:

Cooking Time: 30 minutes

Ingredients:

- 1 tablespoon of olive oil
- 1 onion, chopped
- 2 cloves garlic, minced

- 1 lb. boneless, skinless pork chops, thinly sliced
- 1 cup of chicken broth
- 1/2 cup frozen peas
- 1/4 cup chopped fresh parsley
- Salt and pepper to taste

Instructions:

1. Heat olive oil in a large skillet over medium heat, then add the onion and cook it until softened, about 5 minutes.
2. Stir in the garlic and cook for another minute, until fragrant.
3. Add pork and cook until browned on all sides, about 5-7 minutes.
4. Then pour in chicken broth and boil it. Reduce heat and cook for 10 minutes, or until pork is cooked through.
5. Stir in frozen peas and cook for 2-3 minutes, until heated through.
6. Sprinkle with parsley and season with salt and pepper to taste.
7. Serve over rice or noodles.

Nutritional Value (per serving):

- Calories: 400
- Protein: 30g
- Fat: 20g

- Carbohydrates: 30g
- Fiber: 2g

Tasty Lamb Ribs:

Cooking Time: 2–3 hours (depending on the thickness of the ribs)

Ingredients:

- 2 racks lamb ribs
- 1 tablespoon of olive oil
- 1 teaspoon dried thyme
- 1/2 teaspoon salt
- 1/4 teaspoon black pepper
- 1/4 cup brown sugar
- 1/4 cup apple cider vinegar
- 1 tablespoon Dijon mustard

Instructions:

1. Preheat the oven to 325°F (165°C). Line a baking sheet with foil.
2. In a small bowl, combine the olive oil, thyme, salt, and pepper. Rub the mixture onto the lamb ribs.
3. Place ribs on the prepared baking sheet, meaty side up.
4. In a small saucepan, combine brown sugar, apple cider vinegar, and Dijon mustard.

Bring to a simmer over medium heat, stirring constantly, until the sugar is dissolved.

5. Brush the ribs with the glaze and bake for 30 minutes.
6. Continue to bake, brushing with the glaze every 30 minutes, until ribs are tender and falling off the bone, about 2–3 hours for thick ribs.

Nutritional Value (per serving, 4 ribs):

- Calories: 500
- Protein: 40g
- Fat: 30g
- Carbohydrates: 20g
- Fiber: 1g

Greek Style Lamb Chops:

Cooking Time: 15-20 minutes (including marinating)

Ingredients:

- 8 lamb chops
- 1/4 cup olive oil
- 2 tablespoons of lemon juice
- 1 tablespoon dried oregano
- 1 teaspoon garlic powder

- 1/2 teaspoon salt
- 1/4 teaspoon black pepper

Instructions:

1. Combine olive oil, lemon juice, oregano, garlic powder, salt, and pepper in a bowl. Whisk to blend.
2. Place the lamb chops in the marinade and stir to coat them evenly. Cover and refrigerate for at least 30 minutes, or up to overnight for deeper flavors.
3. Preheat the grill to medium-high heat. Alternatively, heat a large cast-iron skillet over medium-high heat.
4. Remove the lamb chops from the marinade and grill or pan-fry for 3–4 minutes per side, or until cooked to desired doneness.
5. Serve immediately with lemon wedges and your favorite sides.

Nutritional Value (per serving):

- Calories: 350
- Protein: 30g
- Fat: 20g
- Carbohydrates: 1g
- Fiber: 0g
-

Cooking Time: 20 minutes

Ingredients:

- 1 pound of ground beef or sausage
- 1/2 cup chopped onion
- 1/4 cup chopped green pepper
- 2 cloves garlic, minced
- 1/2 teaspoon chili powder
- 1/4 teaspoon cumin
- 1/4 teaspoon paprika
- 1/4 teaspoon salt
- 1/4 teaspoon black pepper
- 1/4 cup of ketchup
- 1/4 cup brown sugar

Instructions:

1. Heat a large skillet over medium heat. Add ground beef or sausage and cook until browned, breaking it up with a spoon.
2. Drain off any excess fat.
3. Add onion, green pepper, and garlic to the skillet and cook until softened, about 5 minutes.
4. Stir in chili powder, cumin, paprika, salt, and pepper. Cook for 1 minute, until fragrant.

5. Stir in ketchup and brown sugar. Bring to a simmer and cook for 5 minutes, stirring occasionally.
6. Let cool slightly before spreading on crackers, bread, or pita bread.

Nutritional Value (per serving, 2 tablespoons):

- Calories: 150
- Protein: 8g
- Fat: 10g
- Carbohydrates: 10g
- Fiber: 1g

3. Pork and Figs Mix:

Cooking Time: 20 minutes

Ingredients:

- 1 tablespoon of olive oil
- 1 onion, chopped
- 2 cloves garlic, minced
- 1 pound boneless, skinless pork loin, thinly sliced
- 8 fresh figs, quartered
- 1/4 cup dry white wine (optional)
- 1/4 cup chicken broth

1 tablespoon chopped fresh thyme

- Salt and pepper to taste

Instructions:

1. Heat olive oil in a large skillet over medium heat. Then add the onion and cook until softened, for about 5 minutes.
2. Stir in the garlic and cook for another minute, until fragrant.
3. Add pork and cook until browned on all sides, about 5-7 minutes.
4. Stir in figs, wine (if using), chicken broth, and thyme. Season with salt and pepper.
5. Bring to a simmer and cook for 5-7 minutes, or until the pork is cooked through and the figs are tender.
6. Serve over rice or couscous.

Nutritional Value (per serving):

- Calories: 400
- Protein: 30g
- Fat: 20g
- Carbohydrates: 25g
- Fiber: 3g

Lemony lamb and potatoes

CHAPTER 6

Flavorful Delights Lunch Recipes

Smoky Red Beans and Rice
(vegetarian):

Cooking Time: 45 minutes (plus soaking time for beans)

Ingredients:

- 1 ½ cups dried kidney beans, soaked overnight and drained
- 1 tablespoon of olive oil
- 1 onion, chopped
- 2 cloves garlic, minced
- 1 green bell pepper, chopped
- 1 red bell pepper, chopped
- 1 teaspoon smoked paprika
- 1/2 teaspoon ground cumin
- 1/4 teaspoon cayenne pepper (optional)
- 4 cups of vegetable broth
- 1 (14.5 oz) can diced tomatoes, undrained
- 1 bay leaf
- 1 cup of cooked brown rice
- Salt and pepper to taste

Instructions:

1. Just heat olive oil over medium heat in a large pot. Cook until softened after adding the onion for about 5 minutes.
2. Stir in garlic, bell peppers, paprika, cumin, and cayenne pepper (if using). Cook for another 5 minutes, until the peppers are softened.
3. Add vegetable broth, diced tomatoes with their juices, bay leaf, and drained beans. Bring to a boil, then reduce heat and simmer for 30 minutes, or until beans are tender.
4. Remove the bay leaf and stir in the cooked brown rice. Season with salt and pepper, to taste.
5. Serve warm, garnished with chopped fresh parsley or cilantro (optional).

Nutritional Value (per serving):

- Calories: 400
- Protein: 15g
- Fat: 10g
- Carbohydrates: 60g
- Fiber: 10g
-

Cooking Time: 30 minutes (including chilling time)

Ingredients:

- 1 pound of raw shrimp, peeled and deveined
- 1 tablespoon of olive oil
- 1/2 teaspoon dried oregano
- 1/4 teaspoon salt
- 1/4 teaspoon black pepper
- 1 cucumber, chopped
- 1 large tomato, chopped
- 1/2 red onion, thinly sliced
- 1/4 cup chopped fresh parsley
- 1/4 cup crumbled feta cheese
- 2 tablespoons of lemon juice
- 1 tablespoon of olive oil

Instructions:

1. In a small bowl, combine olive oil, oregano, salt, and pepper. Toss shrimp with the mixture and marinate for 15 minutes at room temperature.
2. Heat a grill pan or skillet over medium-high heat. Cook for 2-3 minutes per side, or until the shrimp are pink and fully cooked.
3. In a large bowl, combine the cucumber, tomato, red onion, parsley, and feta cheese.

4. Add the cooked shrimp and drizzle with lemon juice and olive oil. Toss to coat.
5. Chill for 30 minutes for the best flavor, and then serve.

Nutritional Value (per serving):

- Calories: 300
- Protein: 30g
- Fat: 10g
- Carbohydrates: 15g
- Fiber: 2g

Baked Balsamic Fish

Ingredients:

- Get 4 white fish fillets (such as tilapia or cod).
- 1/4 cup balsamic vinegar
- 2 tablespoons of olive oil
- 2 cloves garlic, minced
- 1 teaspoon dried oregano
- Salt and pepper to taste
- Lemon wedges for serving

Instructions:

1. Preheat the oven to 375°F (190°C).
2. Then place the fish fillets in a baking dish.

3. In a small bowl, whisk together balsamic vinegar, olive oil, minced garlic, dried oregano, salt, and pepper.
4. Pour the balsamic mixture over the fish, ensuring each fillet is coated.
5. Bake for 15-20 minutes or until the fish flakes easily with a fork.
6. Serve with lemon wedges.

Nutritional Value (per serving):

- Calories: ~200
- Protein: ~25g
- Fat: ~9g
- Carbohydrates: ~2g

Greek Style Quesadillas

Ingredients:

- 4 whole wheat tortillas
- 1 cup cooked chicken, shredded
- 1 cup spinach, chopped
- 1/2 cup feta cheese, crumbled
- 1/4 cup red onion, thinly sliced
- 1/4 cup Kalamata olives, sliced
- 1 teaspoon dried oregano
- Olive oil for cooking

Instructions:

1. In a bowl, mix shredded chicken, spinach, feta cheese, red onion, Kalamata olives, and dried oregano.
2. Place a portion of the mixture on one half of each tortilla, and then fold the other half over, creating a quesadilla.
3. Heat olive oil in a skillet over medium heat.
4. Cook each quesadilla for 2-3 minutes on each side or until golden brown.
5. Slice and serve.

Nutritional Value (per serving):

- Calories: ~350
- Protein: ~20g
- Fat: ~15g
- Carbohydrates: ~30g

Chicken and Cabbage Platter

Ingredients:

- 1 lb. chicken breasts, sliced
- 1 small green cabbage, shredded
- 2 carrots, julienned
- 2 tablespoons of soy sauce
- 1 tablespoon sesame oil
- 1 tablespoon of rice vinegar

- 1 teaspoon ginger, grated
- 2 cloves garlic, minced
- Green onions for garnish

Instructions:

1. Heat a large skillet over medium-high heat. Cook until browned after adding the sliced chicken and cooking through.
2. Add shredded cabbage and julienned carrots to the skillet. Stir-fry until vegetables are tender-crisp.
3. In a small bowl, whisk together soy sauce, sesame oil, rice vinegar, grated ginger, and minced garlic.
4. Pour the sauce over the chicken and vegetables. Stir to combine.
5. Garnish with green onions, and serve.

Nutritional Value (per serving):

- Calories: ~300
- Protein: ~30g
- Fat: ~8g
- Carbohydrates: ~25g

Ingredients:

- 1 lb. ground chicken
- 1 onion, diced
- 2 bell peppers, diced
- 2 cloves garlic, minced
- 1 can (15 oz) of black beans, drained and rinsed
- 1 can (15 oz) diced tomatoes
- 1 cup of chicken broth
- 1 tablespoon chili powder
- 1 teaspoon of cumin
- Salt and pepper to taste
- Greek yogurt and cilantro for garnish

Instructions:

1. In a large pot, cook ground chicken until browned.
2. Add diced onion, bell peppers, and minced garlic. Cook until the vegetables are softened.
3. Stir in black beans, diced tomatoes, chicken broth, chili powder, cumin, salt, and pepper.
4. Simmer for 20–30 minutes, allowing flavors to meld.

5. Serve with a dollop of Greek yogurt, and garnish with cilantro.

Nutritional Value (per serving):

- Calories: ~350
- Protein: ~25g
- Fat: ~10g
- Carbohydrates: ~35g

Scallops with peppers

Ingredients:

- 1 lb. scallops, patted dry
- 1 red bell pepper, thinly sliced
- 1 yellow bell pepper, thinly sliced
- 2 tablespoons of olive oil
- 2 cloves garlic, minced
- 1 teaspoon smoked paprika
- Salt and pepper to taste
- Fresh parsley for garnish

Instructions:

1. You have to heat the olive oil in a skillet over medium-high heat.
2. Add sliced bell peppers and cook until they begin to soften.

3. Add minced garlic and cook for an additional 30 seconds.
4. Push the peppers to the side and add the scallops to the skillet. Just cook for 2-3 minutes per side, or you cook until golden brown.
5. Sprinkle smoked paprika, salt, and pepper over the scallops and peppers. Toss to combine.
6. Garnish with fresh parsley before serving.

Cooking Time: ~10 minutes

Nutritional Value (per serving):

- Calories: ~200
- Protein: ~20g
- Fat: ~10g
- Carbohydrates: ~8g

Mediterranean Chicken

Ingredients:

- 4 boneless, skinless chicken breasts
- 1 lemon, juiced
- 3 tablespoons of olive oil
- 2 teaspoons dried oregano
- 1 teaspoon garlic powder
- Salt and pepper to taste

- Cherry tomatoes and olives for garnish

Instructions:

1. Preheat the oven to 375°F (190°C).
2. In a bowl, mix lemon juice, olive oil, dried oregano, garlic powder, salt, and pepper.
3. Then you place the chicken breasts in a baking dish and pour the marinade over them.
4. Just Bake for 25-30 minutes or until the chicken is fully cooked.
5. Garnish with cherry tomatoes and olives before serving.

Cooking Time: ~30 minutes

Nutritional Value (per serving):

- Calories: ~300
- Protein: ~30g
- Fat: ~15g
- Carbohydrates: ~5g

Garlic Shrimp Pasta

Ingredients:

- 8 oz. linguine or spaghetti
- 1 lb shrimp, peeled and deveined

- 4 tablespoons of butter
- 4 cloves garlic, minced
- 1/2 teaspoon red pepper flakes (optional)
- 1/4 cup chicken broth
- Juice of 1 lemon
- Salt and pepper to taste
- Fresh parsley for garnish

Instructions:

1. Cook pasta according to package instructions.
2. Melt butter over medium heat in a large skillet. Then add minced garlic and red pepper flakes and sauté until fragrant.
3. Add shrimp to the skillet and cook until they turn pink.
4. Pour in chicken broth and lemon juice. Season with salt and pepper.
5. Toss the cooked pasta into the skillet, ensuring it's well coated with the garlic shrimp mixture.
6. Garnish with fresh parsley before serving.

Cooking Time: ~20 minutes

Nutritional Value (per serving):

- Calories: ~400
- Protein: ~25g

- Fat: ~15g
- Carbohydrates: ~40g

Beef and Zucchini Skillet

Ingredients:

- 1 lb. lean ground beef
- 2 zucchinis, diced
- 1 onion, diced
- 2 cloves garlic, minced
- 1 teaspoon Italian seasoning
- Salt and pepper to taste
- 1 cup of tomato sauce
- 1 cup shredded mozzarella cheese
- Fresh basil for garnish

Instructions:

1. In a large skillet, cook ground beef over medium-high heat until browned.
2. Add diced zucchini, onion, and minced garlic. Cook until the vegetables are tender.
3. Season with Italian seasoning, salt, and pepper.
4. Pour the tomato sauce over the beef and vegetables, stirring to combine.
5. Sprinkle shredded mozzarella over the mixture and cover until the cheese melts.
6. Garnish with fresh basil before serving.

Cooking Time: ~20 minutes

Nutritional Value (per serving):

- Calories: ~400
- Protein: ~30g
- Fat: ~20g
- Carbohydrates: ~20g

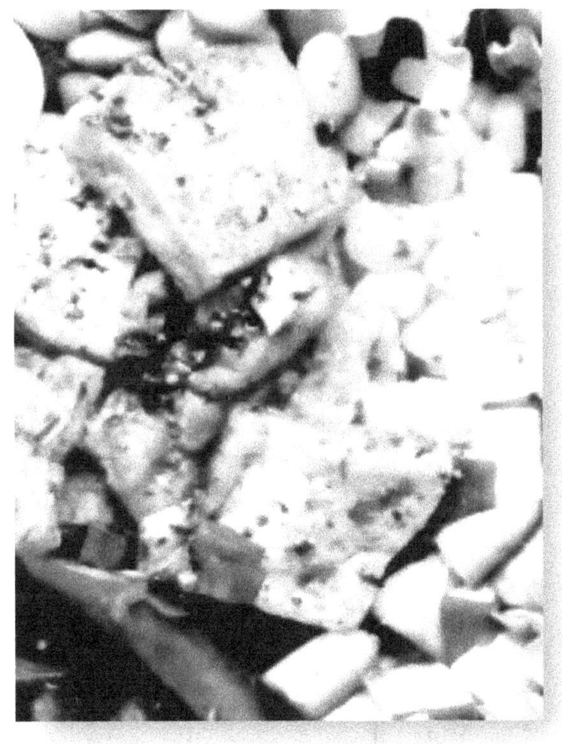

Mouthwatering Dinner Recipes
Salmon Skillet

Ingredients:

- 4 salmon fillets
- 2 tablespoons of olive oil
- 1 lemon, sliced
- 2 cloves garlic, minced
- 1 teaspoon dried dill
- Salt and pepper to taste
- Fresh parsley for garnish

Instructions:

1. Season salmon fillets with salt, pepper, and dried dill.
2. Heat olive oil in a skillet over medium-high heat.
3. Then you add minced garlic and cook until fragrant.
4. Place the salmon fillets in the skillet, skin side down. Then you have to cook for 4-5 minutes per side, or until the salmon flakes easily.

5. Squeeze lemon juice over the salmon and garnish with fresh parsley before serving.

Cooking Time: ~10 minutes

Nutritional Value (per serving):

- Calories: ~300
- Protein: ~30g
- Fat: ~18g
- Carbohydrates: ~2g

Tuna Sandwiches

Ingredients:

- 2 cans (5 oz each) tuna, drained
- 1/4 cup mayonnaise
- 1 celery stalk, finely chopped
- 1 tablespoon Dijon mustard
- Salt and pepper to taste
- Whole wheat bread
- Lettuce and tomato slices for topping

Instructions:

1. In a bowl, mix tuna, mayonnaise, chopped celery, Dijon mustard, salt, and pepper.
2. Toast whole wheat bread slices.

3. Spread the tuna mixture on the bread and top with lettuce and tomato slices.
4. Assemble sandwiches and serve.

Cooking Time: ~15 minutes

Nutritional Value (per serving):

- Calories: ~300
- Protein: ~20g
- Fat: ~15g
- Carbohydrates: ~20g

Steamed Garlic Chicken Breasts

Ingredients:

- 4 boneless, skinless chicken breasts
- 4 cloves garlic, minced
- 2 tablespoons of soy sauce
- 1 tablespoon sesame oil
- 1 teaspoon ginger, grated
- Green onions for garnish

Instructions:

1. Place the chicken breasts in a steamer basket.
2. In a small bowl, mix minced garlic, soy sauce, sesame oil, and grated ginger.

3. Pour the sauce over the chicken breasts.
4. Steam for 15-20 minutes or until the chicken is cooked through.
5. Garnish with chopped green onions before serving.

Cooking Time: ~20 minutes

Nutritional Value (per serving):

- Calories: ~250
- Protein: ~30g
- Fat: ~10g
- Carbohydrates: ~2g

Honey Pork Meatballs

Ingredients:

- 1 lb. ground pork
- 1/4 cup of breadcrumbs
- 2 tablespoons of honey
- 2 tablespoons of soy sauce
- 1 teaspoon garlic powder
- 1/2 teaspoon ground ginger
- Green onions for garnish

Instructions:

1. Preheat the oven to 375°F (190°C).

2. In a bowl, combine the ground pork,
    breadcrumbs, honey, soy sauce, garlic
    powder, and ground ginger.
3. You have to shape the mixture into
    meatballs, and after that, you place them on
    a baking sheet.
4. Bake for 20–25 minutes, or until the
    meatballs are cooked through.
5. Garnish with chopped green onions before
    serving.

Cooking Time: ~25 minutes

Nutritional Value (per serving):

- Calories: ~300
- Protein: ~20g
- Fat: ~20g
- Carbohydrates: ~10g

Cauliflower Risotto

Ingredients:

- 1 cauliflower, riced
- 2 tablespoons of olive oil
- 1 onion, finely chopped
- 2 cloves garlic, minced
- 1/2 cup vegetable broth
- 1/4 cup grated Parmesan cheese

- Salt and pepper to taste
- Fresh parsley for garnish

Instructions:

1. In a food processor, rice the cauliflower.
2. Heat olive oil in a skillet over medium heat. Then add chopped onion and minced garlic to it and cook until softened.
3. Add the raced cauliflower to the skillet and stir.
4. Pour vegetable broth over the cauliflower, cover, and cook for 8–10 minutes or until tender.
5. Stir in Parmesan cheese, salt, and pepper. Garnish with fresh parsley before serving.

Cooking Time: ~15 minutes

Nutritional Value (per serving):

- Calories: ~150
- Protein: ~5g
- Fat: ~10g
- Carbohydrates: ~10g

Ingredients:

- Just get 1 lb. boneless, skinless chicken thighs, cut into bite-sized pieces.
- 1/4 cup soy sauce
- 2 tablespoons of mirin
- 1 tablespoon of honey
- 1 tablespoon of sake (optional)
- 2 cloves garlic, minced
- 1 teaspoon grated ginger
- Green onions for garnish
- Sesame seeds for garnish

Instructions:

1. In a bowl, mix soy sauce, mirin, honey, sake, minced garlic, and grated ginger to make the marinade.
2. Thread chicken pieces onto skewers.
3. Brush the chicken skewers with the marinade.
4. Grill or broil the chicken skewers for 8–10 minutes or until fully cooked.
5. Garnish with chopped green onions and sesame seeds before serving.

Cooking Time: ~10 minutes

Nutritional Value (per serving):

- Calories: ~200
- Protein: ~20g
- Fat: ~10g
- Carbohydrates: ~10g

Spicy Salmon

Ingredients:

- 4 salmon fillets
- 2 tablespoons of olive oil
- 1 teaspoon chili powder
- 1/2 teaspoon cayenne pepper
- 1 teaspoon paprika
- 1 teaspoon garlic powder
- Salt and pepper to taste
- Lemon wedges for serving

Instructions:

1. Preheat the oven to 400°F (200°C).
2. Place salmon fillets on a baking sheet.
3. In a small bowl, mix olive oil, chili powder, cayenne pepper, paprika, garlic powder, salt, and pepper.
4. Brush the spicy mixture over the salmon fillets.

5. Bake for 12–15 minutes or until the salmon flakes easily with a fork.
6. Serve with lemon wedges.

Cooking Time: ~15 minutes

Nutritional Value (per serving):

- Calories: ~300
- Protein: ~25g
- Fat: ~20g
- Carbohydrates: ~2g

Steak with Vegetables

Ingredients:

- 2 sirloin steaks
- 2 tablespoons of olive oil
- 1 teaspoon dried thyme
- 1 teaspoon garlic powder
- Salt and pepper to taste
- 1 zucchini, sliced
- 1 bell pepper, sliced
- 1 red onion, sliced

Instructions:

1. You have to preheat the grill or a grill pan over medium-high heat.

2. Rub steaks with olive oil, dried thyme, garlic powder, salt, and pepper.
3. Grill steaks to your desired doneness (about 4-5 minutes per side for medium-rare).
4. In a separate pan, sauté zucchini, bell pepper, and red onion until tender.
5. Serve the grilled steaks over the sautéed vegetables.

Cooking Time: ~10 minutes

Nutritional Value (per serving):

- Calories: ~400
- Protein: ~30g
- Fat: ~25g
- Carbohydrates: ~10g

Citrus-Baked Fish

Ingredients:

- Get 4 white fish fillets (such as tilapia or cod).
- 2 tablespoons of olive oil
- 1 orange, juiced
- 1 lemon, juiced
- 2 cloves garlic, minced
- 1 teaspoon dried thyme
- Salt and pepper to taste

- Fresh parsley for garnish

Instructions:

1. Preheat the oven to 375°F (190°C).
2. Then you place the fish fillets in a baking dish.
3. In a bowl, whisk together olive oil, orange juice, lemon juice, minced garlic, dried thyme, salt, and pepper.
4. Pour the citrus mixture over the fish.
5. Bake for 15-20 minutes or until the fish flakes easily with a fork.
6. Garnish with fresh parsley before serving.

Cooking Time: ~20 minutes

Nutritional Value (per serving):

- Calories: ~250
- Protein: ~20g
- Fat: ~15g
- Carbohydrates: ~5g

Kale and Tuna Bowl

Ingredients:

- 4 cups kale, chopped
- 1 can (5 oz) tuna, drained

- 1 cup cherry tomatoes, halved
- 1/2 cucumber, sliced
- 1/4 cup feta cheese, crumbled
- 2 tablespoons of olive oil
- 1 tablespoon balsamic vinegar
- Salt and pepper to taste
- Pumpkin seeds for garnish (optional)

Instructions:

1. In a bowl, combine chopped kale, drained tuna, cherry tomatoes, cucumber, and crumbled feta cheese.
2. In a small bowl, whisk together olive oil, balsamic vinegar, salt, and pepper.
3. Pour the dressing over the kale and tuna mixture and toss to combine.
4. Garnish with pumpkin seeds, if desired.

Cooking Time: ~10 minutes

Nutritional Value (per serving):

- Calories: ~350
- Protein: ~25g
- Fat: ~20g
- Carbohydrates: ~15g

Ingredients:

- 2 cups of spinach leaves
- 1 cucumber, peeled and chopped
- 1 green apple, cored and sliced
- 1 lemon, peeled
- 1-inch piece of ginger, peeled
- 1 cup of water or coconut water
- Ice cubes (optional)

Instructions:

1. Place all the ingredients in a blender.
2. Blend until smooth.
3. Then, to extract the juice, strain the mixture.
4. Serve over ice, if desired.

Preparation Time: ~10 minutes

Nutritional Value (per serving):

- Calories: ~50
- Fiber: ~5g
- Vitamin A: ~100% DV

- Vitamin C: ~50% DV

Blue Breeze Shake

Ingredients:

- 1 cup blueberries (fresh or frozen)
- 1 banana
- 1/2 cup Greek yogurt
- 1/2 cup almond milk
- 1 tablespoon of chia seeds
- Ice cubes (optional)

Instructions:

1. Place all the ingredients in a blender.
2. Blend until smooth.
3. If a colder consistency is desired, you can add ice cubes.

Preparation Time: ~5 minutes

Nutritional Value (per serving):

- Calories: ~250
- Protein: ~10g
- Fiber: ~8g
- Calcium: ~15% DV
-

Ingredients:

- 1 green tea bag (brewed and cooled)
- 1 cup of spinach leaves
- 1/2 cucumber, peeled and sliced
- 1 kiwi, peeled and sliced
- 1 tablespoon of honey
- Ice cubes (optional)

Instructions:

1. Brew green tea and let it cool.
2. Place all the ingredients in a blender.
3. Blend until smooth.
4. Add ice cubes, if desired.

Preparation Time: ~8 minutes

Nutritional Value (per serving):

- Calories: ~80
- Antioxidants: High
- Vitamin K: ~100% DV

Ingredients:

- 1 cup of red grapes
- 1 peach, pitted and sliced
- 1/2 cup plain yogurt
- 1/2 cup of orange juice
- 1 tablespoon flaxseeds
- Ice cubes (optional)

Instructions:

1. Place all the ingredients in a blender.
2. Blend until smooth.
3. If a colder consistency is desired, you can add ice cubes.

Preparation Time: ~7 minutes

Nutritional Value (per serving):

- Calories: ~150
- Fiber: ~5g
- Vitamin C: ~60% DV

Ingredients:

- 1 cup watermelon, cubed
- 1/2 cup pineapple chunks
- 1/2 cucumber, sliced
- 1 tablespoon of lime juice
- 1 tablespoon of mint leaves
- Ice cubes (optional)

Instructions:

1. Place all the ingredients in a blender.
2. Blend until smooth.
3. Add ice cubes, if desired.

Preparation Time: ~6 minutes

Nutritional Value (per serving):

- Calories: ~50
- Hydration: High
- Vitamin A: ~20% DV

Ingredients:

- 1 cucumber, peeled and chopped
- 1 green apple, cored and sliced
- 1 tablespoon grated ginger
- 1 cup of coconut water
- 1 tablespoon of chia seeds
- Ice cubes (optional)

Instructions:

1. Place all the ingredients in a blender.
2. Blend until smooth.
3. Add ice cubes, if desired.

Preparation Time: ~8 minutes

Nutritional Value (per serving):

- Calories: ~70
- Fiber: ~6g
- Anti-Inflammatory: High

CHAPTER 9

Chicken and Carrot Stew:

- o **Cooking Time:** 1 hour
- o **Ingredients:**
    - 1.5 lbs chicken thighs, boneless and skinless
    - 1 cup carrots, sliced
    - 1 onion, diced
    - 2 cloves garlic, minced
    - 4 cups of chicken broth
    - 1 cup potatoes, diced
    - Salt and pepper to taste
- o **Instructions:**

1. In a large pot, sauté onions and garlic until translucent.
2. Add chicken thighs and brown them on all sides.
3. Add carrots, potatoes, and chicken broth.
4. Season with salt and pepper.
5. Simmer for 45 minutes to 1 hour, or until the chicken is cooked through.

- o **Nutritional Value:** (per serving)

  - Calories: 300
  - Protein: 25g
  - Carbohydrates: 20g
  - Fat: 12g

Fajita Soup:

- o **Cooking Time:** 45 minutes
- o **Ingredients:**
  - 1 lb. chicken breast, thinly sliced
  - 1 bell pepper, sliced
  - 1 onion, sliced
  - 2 cloves garlic, minced
  - 1 can black beans, drained
  - 1 can of diced tomatoes
  - 4 cups of chicken broth
  - 1 teaspoon of cumin
  - 1 teaspoon chili powder
- o **Instructions:**

  1. Sauté the chicken, bell pepper, onion, and garlic until the chicken is browned.
  2. Add black beans, diced tomatoes, chicken broth, cumin, and chili powder.

3. Simmer for 30 minutes.
- o **Nutritional Value:** (per serving)

  - Calories: 280
  - Protein: 30g
  - Carbohydrates: 25g
  - Fat: 8g

Rotisserie Chicken Noodle Soup:

- o **Cooking Time:** 1 hour
- o **Ingredients:**
  - 1 rotisserie chicken, shredded
  - 8 cups of chicken broth
  - 2 carrots, sliced
  - 2 celery stalks, sliced
  - 1 onion, diced
  - 1 cup of egg noodles
  - Salt and pepper to taste
- o **Instructions:**

  1. In a pot, combine chicken broth, carrots, celery, and onion. Bring to a boil.
  2. Add the egg noodles and simmer until the vegetables are tender.
  3. Stir in the shredded rotisserie chicken.

4. Season with salt and pepper.

o **Nutritional Value:** (per serving)

- Calories: 350
- Protein: 28g
- Carbohydrates: 30g
- Fat: 12g

Sweetcorn Soup:

o **Cooking Time:** 30 minutes
o **Ingredients:**
- 2 cups sweetcorn kernels
- 4 cups of chicken or vegetable broth
- 1 cup heavy cream
- 1 tablespoon of butter
- Salt and pepper to taste

o **Instructions:**

1. Blend half of the sweetcorn with 2 cups of broth until smooth.
2. In a pot, melt the butter and add the remaining sweetcorn.

3. Pour in the blended mixture,
   the rest of the broth, and
   heavy cream.
4. Simmer for 15–20 minutes.
5. Season with salt and pepper.

- **Nutritional Value:** (per serving)

  - Calories: 250
  - Protein: 5g
  - Carbohydrates: 30g
  - Fat: 15g

Yucatan Chicken Lime Soup:

- **Cooking Time:** 45 minutes
- **Ingredients:**
  - 1 lb chicken thighs, boneless, skinless
  - 1 onion, finely chopped
  - 2 cloves garlic, minced
  - 2 tomatoes, diced
  - 4 cups of chicken broth
  - 2 limes, juiced
  - 1 teaspoon of cumin
  - 1 teaspoon of oregano
  - Salt and pepper to taste

- o **Instructions:**

    1. In a pot, cook chicken, onion, and garlic until the chicken is browned.
    2. Add tomatoes, chicken broth, lime juice, cumin, and oregano.
    3. Simmer for 30 minutes.
    4. Season with salt and pepper.

- o **Nutritional Value:** (per serving)

    - Calories: 280
    - Protein: 25g
    - Carbohydrates: 15g
    - Fat: 12g

Roasted Garlic Soup:

- o **Cooking Time:** 1 hour
- o **Ingredients:**
    - 2 heads of garlic
    - 2 tablespoons of olive oil
    - 1 onion, chopped
    - 4 cups of vegetable broth
    - 1 potato, diced
    - 1 cup heavy cream
    - Salt and pepper to taste
- o **Instructions:**

1. Roast garlic heads in the oven with olive oil until the cloves are soft.
2. Sauté the onion in a pot until translucent.
3. Add roasted garlic, vegetable broth, and diced potato.
4. Simmer until the potato is tender.
5. Blend the soup until smooth, and stir in heavy cream.
6. Season with salt and pepper.

- **Nutritional Value:** (per serving)

  - Calories: 320
  - Protein: 5g
  - Carbohydrates: 20g
  - Fat: 25g

Day 1:

Breakfast: It should be scrambled eggs, topped with spinach and whole-grain toast.

Lunch should be grilled chicken salad; eat it with mixed veggies.

Dinner: Baked salmon with quinoa and steamed broccoli

Snack: Greek yogurt with berries

Day 2:

Breakfast: Oatmeal with Banana and Almond Butter

Lunch: Turkey and avocado wrap with a side of carrot sticks

Dinner: You should eat stir-fried tofu with brown rice and assorted vegetables.

Snack: A handful of mixed nuts

Day 3:

Breakfast: Smoothie with kale, banana, Greek yogurt, and chia seeds

Lunch: Quinoa bowl with black beans, corn, and salsa

Dinner: Lemon herb grilled shrimp with sweet potato wedges

Snack: apple slices with peanut butter

Day 4:

Breakfast: whole-grain pancakes with maple syrup and strawberries

Lunch: You will eat chickpeas and vegetable curry, then basmati rice.

Dinner: Baked chicken breast eat with roasted Brussels sprouts and quinoa

Snack: Cottage cheese with pineapple chunks

Day 5:

Breakfast: avocado toast with poached eggs

Lunch will be lentil soup, eaten with a side of whole-grain crackers.

Dinner: Beef stir-fry with broccoli and brown rice

Snack: A handful of cherry tomatoes with mozzarella

Day 6:

Breakfast: Greek yogurt parfait with granola and mixed berries

Lunch: Caprese salad with grilled chicken

Dinner: You will eat baked cod with asparagus and wild rice.

Snack: Hummus with cucumber slices

Day 7:

Breakfast: spinach and feta omelet with whole-grain toast

Lunch: There will be quinoa salad. Eat it with cucumber, tomato, and feta.

Dinner: Vegetable lasagna with a side of green beans

Snack: mixed fruit bowl

Weeks 3 and 4:

Repeat the Week 1 and 2 meal plans.

Weeks 5 and 6:

Day 1:

Breakfast: Overnight oats with almond milk, chia seeds, and sliced peaches

Lunch: Turkey and cranberry wrap with a side of baby carrots

Dinner: Grilled swordfish with quinoa and roasted asparagus

Snack: Cottage cheese with sliced Kiwi

Day 2:

Breakfast: Whole-grain waffles with yogurt and blueberries

Lunch: Chickpea salad; eat it with tomatoes, cucumbers, and feta.

Dinner: Shrimp and broccoli stir-fry with brown rice

Snack: A handful of almonds

Day 3:

Breakfast: smoked salmon bagel with cream cheese and capers

Lunch: Lentil and vegetable stir-fry with quinoa

Dinner: Baked chicken thighs with sweet potato mash and green beans

Snack: Greek yogurt with honey

Day 4:

Breakfast: banana walnut muffins with a side of mixed berries

Lunch: It will be quinoa and black bean-stuffed bell peppers.

Dinner: Turkey meatballs with whole-grain spaghetti and marinara sauce

Snack: sliced pear with cheese

Day 5:

Breakfast: veggie omelet with whole-grain toast

Lunch: spinach and strawberry salad with grilled chicken

Dinner: Grilled tilapia with lemon and dill, accompanied by quinoa

Snack: Hummus with carrot sticks

Day 6:

Breakfast: Smoothie bowl with mango, pineapple, and granola

Lunch: Quinoa and roasted vegetable wrap

Dinner: Baked cod with lemon and herbs, served with wild rice

Snack: mixed nuts and dried fruits

Day 7:

Breakfast: avocado and tomato toast with poached eggs

Lunch: Caprese quinoa salad with grilled shrimp

Dinner: Vegetable stir-fry with tofu and brown rice

Snack: apple slices with almond butter

Week 7 & 8:

Repeat week 5& 6 meal plan

Good Exercise That Will Help Heal Your Fatty Liver

Aerobic Exercises:

Brisk Walking: Strive for at least 30 minutes of brisk walking most days of the week. Begin at a moderate pace and progressively build intensity.

Cycling has cardiovascular advantages, whether done outdoors or on a stationary bike.

Strength Training:

Bodyweight exercises, such as squats, lunges, and push-ups, can help you improve muscle strength.

Strength training involves using resistance bands or modest weights. Concentrate on key muscular groups, such as the legs, arms, and core.

Yoga and Flexibility Exercises:

Yoga: Participate in yoga sessions to improve your flexibility, balance, and overall wellbeing.

Stretching: Use mild stretching activities to increase flexibility and minimize muscle tightness.

Interval Training:

High-Intensity Interval Training (HIIT) involves short bursts of intensive activity followed by rest intervals. This can assist boost metabolism and burn calories more efficiently.

Swimming:

Swimming is a low-impact exercise that works the entire body while having minimal stress on the joints. It's an excellent choice for individuals seeking low-impact exercises.

Pilates:

Pilates focuses on core strength, which may be good for those with fatty liver disease.

Tai chi:

Mind-Body Exercise: Tai Chi blends gentle motions, meditation, and deep breathing to promote general wellness.

Stability Ball Exercises:

Balance Training: Use a stability ball to perform exercises that improve balance and stability.

Important considerations:

Gradual Progression: Begin with low-to-moderate intensity and gradually rise as your fitness improves.

Consistency: Aim for frequent, consistent activity, preferably on most days of the week.

Consultation with Healthcare Provider: Always consult with your healthcare provider before beginning a new fitness routine.

Dear Readers,

Heartfelt thanks for choosing "The Fatty Liver Cookbook." Your support is invaluable. I hope the recipes and insights within empower you on your journey to better liver health. Your commitment to well-being is truly appreciated. Happy cooking and living well!